UNDERSTANDING

CHIA SEEDS

AND BENEFITS

A Comprehensive Guide to Health, Nutrition, Focus, Exploring Their Targets, and the Myriad Benefits for a Vibrant Life

DR. LACEY MICHELLE

Disclaimer:

The information provided in this book is for general informational purposes only and is not intended as medical advice.

Readers are encouraged to consult with a qualified healthcare professional for any health concerns or questions.

The author of this book is not affiliated with any individual, website, organization, or products mentioned within.

This book does not endorse or promote any specific brands, services, or external entities. Any references made are purely for illustrative purposes and should not be construed as endorsements.

Readers are responsible for their own decisions and should conduct their own research before making any health-related choices.

Any liability resulting from the use of this information, whether direct or indirect, is disclaimed by the author and publisher.

Contents

About This Book

Chia Seeds - A Nutritional Powerhouse In the opening chapter of "Chia Seeds - A Supplemental Powerhouse," we delve into the impressive nutritional profile of chia seeds. Discover the essential vitamins, minerals, and antioxidants that make chia seeds a super food. We'll explore the numerous health benefits associated with chia seeds, comparing them to other popular superfoods.

History and Cultural Significance

takes us on a journey through time to explore the historical and cultural significance of chia seeds.

Learn about the ancient civilizations that first cultivated these tiny seeds and their role in indigenous cultures. We'll also uncover the resurgence of chia seeds in modern times.

Growing and Harvesting Chia Seeds Understanding the cultivation and farming practices of chia seeds is essential, provides insights into their growth and harvesting. We'll discuss sustainable farming methods, offering a glimpse into the environmentally friendly aspects of chia farming.

Culinary Uses and Recipes For those eager to incorporate chia seeds into their daily diet, offers guidance. From chia puddings and smoothies to savory dishes and baking, you'll find a variety of creative recipes to explore the culinary potential of chia seeds.

Chia Seeds in Health and Wellness

 we delve into the role of chia seeds in health and wellness. Discover how chia seeds can assist in weight management, support digestive health, and enhance the performance of athletes and fitness enthusiasts.

Chia Seeds in Beauty and Skincare Chia seeds aren't just for consumption; they have a place in beauty and skincare too.

Explores their natural beauty benefits, including DIY face masks and scrubs, as well as the use of chia oil for hair and skin.

Chia Seeds in Traditional Medicine Uncover the ancient wisdom surrounding chia seeds in which explores their place in traditional healing practices. We'll also delve into the medicinal properties of chia seeds, backed by modern scientific research.

Sustainability and Ethical Sourcing Chia seeds have an environmental impact, and discusses the importance of sustainable chia seed farming and ethical sourcing initiatives. Learn how conscientious choices can benefit both the environment and local communities.

Chia Seeds in Popular Culture Chia seeds have transcended their dietary utility to become a part of popular culture. In this chapter, we explore their rise in popularity, their presence in literature, art, and media, and the "Chia Seed Revolution" that has taken the world by storm.

Conclusion As we conclude our journey through the world of chia seeds, readers will have gained a holistic understanding of the nutritional, cultural, culinary, and wellness aspects of these remarkable seeds.

Whether you're looking to enhance your health, beauty, or overall well-being, "Chia

Seeds - A Supplemental Powerhouse" is your comprehensive guide to harnessing the potential of chia seeds.

CHAPTER ONE

Nutritional Value Of Chia Seeds

Chia seeds, scientifically known as Salvia hispanica, have gained immense popularity in recent years as a superfood due to their impressive nutritional profile.

These tiny seeds, native to Central America, have been consumed for centuries and were even used as a staple food by ancient civilizations like the Aztecs and Mayans. Chia seeds are packed with essential nutrients, making them a valuable addition to a well-balanced diet.

Chia Seeds' Nutrient Profile

Chia seeds are renowned for their exceptional nutrient density. These seeds are an excellent source of several key nutrients, including dietary fiber, protein, healthy fats, vitamins, and minerals. One of the standout features of chia seeds is their high content of alpha-linolenic acid (ALA), a form of omega-3 fatty acid. Just one ounce of chia seeds can provide a significant portion of the recommended daily intake of ALA. Moreover, chia seeds are rich in fiber, with a significant proportion of it being soluble fiber. This fiber content can aid in digestive health and help with feelings of fullness, making them a valuable addition to weight management and overall well-being.

Additionally, chia seeds are packed with antioxidants, such as quercetin and chlorogenic acid, which can help combat oxidative stress and reduce the risk of chronic diseases. Chia seeds are also a good source of essential minerals like calcium, magnesium, phosphorus, and manganese, which are crucial for bone health and various metabolic processes in the body.

The Role Of Chia Seeds In A Healthy Diet
Chia seeds offer various health benefits when incorporated into a balanced diet. One of the most prominent advantages is their role in heart health. The high omega-3 fatty acid content, primarily ALA, can help reduce the risk of heart disease by lowering levels of "bad" LDL cholesterol and triglycerides while increasing "good" HDL cholesterol. The soluble fiber in chia seeds also contributes to heart health by regulating blood pressure and preventing inflammation.

Moreover, chia seeds are an excellent choice for individuals with diabetes or those looking to manage blood sugar levels. The soluble fiber in chia seeds can slow down the absorption of sugars in the bloodstream, promoting stable blood sugar levels and reducing the risk of spikes and crashes.

Chia seeds can also be a valuable addition to a weight management plan. The combination of protein, fiber, and healthy fats in these seeds promotes feelings of fullness, which can help curb overeating and snacking between meals. This can be particularly useful for those looking to lose weight or maintain a healthy body weight.

Incorporating chia seeds into your diet can also support bone health due to their calcium and phosphorus content. These minerals are essential for maintaining strong bones and preventing conditions like osteoporosis.

Comparing Chia Seeds To Other Superfoods

Chia seeds are often compared to other superfoods like flaxseeds, hemp seeds, and quinoa. While each of these superfoods has its unique nutritional benefits, chia seeds stand out in several ways.

One of the key differentiators is their high ALA content, making them one of the best plant-based sources of omega-3 fatty acids. Flaxseeds are another source of ALA but have a slightly different nutrient profile.

Hemp seeds, on the other hand, are rich in protein and healthy fats, making them an excellent choice for those seeking to boost their protein intake.

However, chia seeds offer a more diverse nutrient profile, including a higher fiber content. Quinoa is another superfood known for its protein content, but it lacks the same omega-3 fatty acids found in chia seeds.

chia seeds are a nutritional powerhouse with a unique blend of essential nutrients, including omega-3 fatty acids, fiber, antioxidants, and minerals.

Their role in promoting heart health, blood sugar regulation, weight management, and bone health makes them a versatile and valuable addition to a healthy diet.

When compared to other superfoods, chia seeds offer distinct advantages, making them a standout choice for those looking to enhance their overall nutritional intake.

Health Benefits Of Chia Seeds

Chia seeds have gained immense popularity in recent years due to their numerous health benefits.

These tiny seeds, derived from the Salvia hispanica plant, pack a powerful nutritional punch and are known for their versatility in various culinary applications. Let's delve into the extensive health benefits of chia seeds across different aspects of well-being.

Weight Management And Chia Seeds

One of the most celebrated aspects of chia seeds is their potential contribution to weight management. Chia seeds are high in dietary fiber, which can promote a feeling of fullness and reduce overall calorie intake. When consumed with fluids, chia seeds can absorb several times their weight in water, forming a gel-like substance in the stomach. This gel can slow down digestion, helping to control appetite and curb snacking. Moreover, the fiber in chia seeds aids in regular bowel movements, which can further support weight management and overall digestive health.

CHAPTER TWO

Digestive Health And Chia Seeds

Chia seeds are renowned for their role in promoting digestive health. The high fiber content in these seeds can help prevent constipation and support a healthy gastrointestinal system.

Chia seeds are a source of both soluble and insoluble fiber, which can regulate bowel movements, reduce the risk of diverticulitis, and maintain a healthy gut microbiome. They also contain a beneficial type of soluble fiber called mucilage, which can soothe and protect the lining of the colon.

Chia Seeds And Heart Health

Consuming chia seeds regularly may contribute to heart health by helping to lower cholesterol levels. The omega-3 fatty acids found in chia seeds, particularly alpha-linolenic acid (ALA), can reduce the risk of cardiovascular diseases by decreasing inflammation, lowering blood pressure, and improving cholesterol profiles. Chia seeds are also packed with antioxidants, which can protect the heart from oxidative stress and reduce the risk of atherosclerosis.

Chia Seeds And Blood Sugar Control

Chia seeds are an excellent choice for individuals seeking to manage their blood sugar levels.

They have a low glycemic index and can help stabilize blood sugar by slowing the digestion and absorption of carbohydrates.

The soluble fiber in chia seeds forms a gel-like barrier that can prevent rapid spikes in blood sugar after meals. This is particularly beneficial for individuals with diabetes or those at risk of developing the condition.

Chia Seeds And Bone Health

Chia seeds are a valuable source of several essential minerals, including calcium, phosphorus, and magnesium.

 These minerals are crucial for maintaining strong and healthy bones. Calcium, in particular, is vital for bone density and skeletal integrity.

Incorporating chia seeds into your diet can help support bone health, especially for individuals who are lactose intolerant or have dietary restrictions that limit their calcium intake.

Chia Seeds And Brain Function

The omega-3 fatty acids in chia seeds, particularly ALA, play a role in maintaining optimal brain function.

These essential fats are important for cognitive development and function. They support brain cell structure, reduce inflammation in the brain, and may help protect against neurodegenerative diseases.

While chia seeds contain a lower amount of omega-3s compared to fatty fish, they can still contribute to overall brain health when included as part of a balanced diet.

Skin And Hair Benefits Of Chia Seeds

Chia seeds offer a range of benefits for skin and hair health. The antioxidants in chia seeds help combat free radicals and oxidative stress, contributing to a youthful and radiant complexion.

Additionally, the omega-3 fatty acids can promote healthy, lustrous hair and reduce scalp dryness and inflammation. Chia seeds can also be used topically in masks and scrubs to exfoliate and moisturize the skin.

Chia seeds are a nutritional powerhouse with a plethora of health benefits. Whether you're looking to manage your weight, improve digestive health, support heart health, control blood sugar, maintain strong bones, enhance brain function, or boost your skin and hair, chia seeds can be a valuable addition to your diet.

Incorporating them into your daily meals and snacks is a convenient and delicious way to reap these health benefits.

CHAPTER THREE

How To Incorporate Chia Seeds Into Your Diet

Chia seeds have gained immense popularity in recent years due to their impressive nutritional profile and versatile culinary applications.

These tiny seeds are packed with fiber, protein, healthy fats, and various essential vitamins and minerals. Incorporating chia seeds into your diet is not only a simple way to boost your nutritional intake but also adds a delightful texture to a wide range of dishes. In this discussion, we will explore different ways to seamlessly integrate chia seeds into your daily meals.

Chia Seeds As A Cooking Ingredient

Chia seeds can be used as a cooking ingredient in a multitude of recipes. Their ability to absorb liquid and form a gel-like consistency makes them an excellent substitute for traditional binders in recipes, like eggs or flour.

Chia seeds can be used to thicken soups, stews, and sauces, making them heartier and more nutritious. Additionally, you can create chia seed "eggs" by mixing chia seeds with water, which is a vegan-friendly alternative to baking. Their mild, nutty flavor complements a variety of dishes, enhancing both texture and nutrition.

Chia Seeds In Smoothies And Drinks

One of the most popular ways to enjoy chia seeds is by adding them to smoothies and beverages. Chia seeds can absorb up to ten times their weight in liquid, forming a gel-like texture. This property is especially useful in creating thicker and more filling smoothies.

Simply mix chia seeds with your favorite liquid, such as almond milk, yogurt, or fruit juice, and let them sit for a while to thicken the drink. The result is a creamy, nutrient-packed beverage that keeps you feeling full and satisfied.

Chia Seeds In Baking And Desserts

Chia seeds are a fantastic addition to baked goods and desserts. You can incorporate them into your recipes by either using chia seed gel or grinding the seeds into a fine powder. Chia seed gel can replace traditional eggs, making your baked goods vegan-friendly and providing an extra dose of omega-3 fatty acids. Chia powder can be added to cookie dough, muffin batter, or even sprinkled on top of cakes and brownies, imparting a subtle crunch and enhancing the nutritional value of your sweet treats.

Chia Seeds In Salads And Side Dishes

Chia seeds can also be sprinkled onto salads and used as a topping for various side dishes. They provide a delightful crunch and a subtle, nutty flavor that pairs well with leafy greens and other ingredients.

You can create a chia seed vinaigrette by blending it with olive oil, vinegar, and your choice of herbs and spices. This vinaigrette not only adds a unique texture but also boosts the nutritional content of your salads, transforming them into a more satisfying and healthful meal.

CHAPTER FOUR

Chia Seed Gel And Its Culinary Uses

Chia seed gel is a versatile culinary tool that can be used in numerous ways. To make chia seed gel, just combine chia seeds with water or another liquid and leave it to sit for a bit, stirring regularly until it forms a gel-like consistency.

This gel can be used as a binding ingredient in recipes, comparable to eggs, or as a thickener in foods like puddings, oats, and yogurt parfaits.

It not only enriches the texture of your foods but also contributes to their nutritional content by supplying fiber, omega-3 fatty acids, and other critical nutrients.

chia seeds are a flexible and healthful addition to your diet. Whether you choose to use them as a cooking ingredient, blend them into smoothies, incorporate them into baking and desserts, sprinkle them on salads and side dishes, or create chia seed gel, these tiny seeds can easily elevate the flavor and nutritional value of your meals while introducing a unique texture to your dishes. So, try including chia seeds into your regular diet to experience its myriad health benefits and culinary delights.

Chia Seeds In Special Diets

Chia seeds have gained enormous popularity in recent years due to their outstanding nutritional content and adaptability. They have become a staple in numerous special diets, delivering a plethora of benefits to those with certain dietary limitations and preferences. Chia seeds are naturally gluten-free, making them an acceptable alternative for persons with gluten sensitivities or those following a gluten-free diet. Their special qualities also make them a great supplement to vegan and vegetarian diets. Furthermore, chia seeds have earned a unique position in the nutrition programs of athletes and fitness fanatics, owing to their capacity to increase performance and help recovery.

Additionally, chia seeds can be a significant component of ketogenic diets, helping individuals fulfill their dietary objectives while enjoying a plethora of health perks.

Chia Seeds In Gluten-Free Diets

One of the biggest attractions of chia seeds for persons on gluten-free diets is their intrinsic lack of gluten.

This protein, found in wheat, barley, and rye, can produce severe effects in people with celiac disease or non-celiac gluten sensitivity.

Chia seeds provide a nutritious and adaptable alternative, allowing those with gluten limitations to incorporate them into their diet safely.

Chia seeds are abundant in dietary fiber, which is commonly missing in gluten-free diets due to the absence of wheat products. This fiber level promotes digestion and helps persons maintain regular bowel movements, a typical concern for those with gluten sensitivities.

Furthermore, chia seeds offer a source of critical nutrients, including omega-3 fatty acids, antioxidants, and minerals like calcium and magnesium. These elements can be lacking in gluten-free diets, making chia seeds a helpful addition to ensure individuals receive a balanced assortment of vitamins and minerals.

Chia seeds can be used in gluten-free baking, substituting typical binders like xanthan gum and eggs while offering a nutritional boost to recipes.

Overall, chia seeds are a terrific resource for individuals adhering to gluten-free diets, bringing both taste and health advantages.

Chia Seeds In Vegan And Vegetarian Diets

Chia seeds have become a valued ingredient in vegan and vegetarian diets due to their high nutritional profile and adaptability.

These diets emphasize plant-based nutrition and chia seeds accord wonderfully with this idea. Chia seeds are a good source of plant-based protein, supplying all essential amino acids, making them an ideal alternative for vegans and vegetarians trying to meet their protein requirements.

They also include a considerable quantity of dietary fiber, which can assist in maintaining digestive health and produce a sensation of fullness.

The omega-3 fatty acids included in chia seeds are another key advantage for people following plant-based diets.

These healthful fats are often linked with fish, but chia seeds provide a good option for receiving omega-3s.

Omega-3s are critical for heart and brain health, and chia seeds assist vegans and vegetarians in maintaining a balanced intake of these essential minerals.

Chia seeds can be used in a wide range of plant-based recipes, such as smoothies, overnight oats, chia puddings, and even as an egg substitute in baking, making them a versatile and nutritious addition to vegan and vegetarian diets.

CHAPTER FIVE

Chia Seeds For Athletes And Fitness Enthusiasts

Chia seeds have earned a unique position in the nutrition regimens of athletes and fitness fanatics, mostly due to their capacity to increase performance and aid in post-workout recovery.

These small seeds are a powerhouse of nutrients that give continuous energy, making them a great choice for pre-and post-workout nourishment. Chia seeds are rich in carbs, particularly in the form of complex carbohydrates, which are released slowly into the bloodstream. This constant flow of energy can assist athletes in maintaining endurance and stamina over longer training sessions.

Moreover, chia seeds are a fantastic source of protein, important for muscle repair and growth. The amino acids included in chia seeds assist in the formation of lean muscle mass and facilitate the healing process after strenuous physical activity. Their high fiber content aids in digestion and helps maintain a healthy gut, which is vital for nutritional absorption and overall well-being.

The hydration effects of chia seeds are also remarkable for athletes. When combined with water, chia seeds generate a gel-like consistency that can assist in retaining hydration during exercise. This gel can slow down the absorption of carbs, helping to maintain blood sugar levels and prevent energy crashes. In summary, chia seeds are a useful tool for athletes and fitness enthusiasts, giving a balanced combination of carbohydrates, protein, healthy fats, and hydration assistance.

Chia Seeds In Ketogenic Diets

Ketogenic diets are characterized by their low carbohydrate, high-fat, and moderate-protein content, aimed to produce a state of ketosis in the body. Chia seeds, with their particular nutritional composition, can be used in ketogenic diets while adhering to tight carbohydrate limitations.

Chia seeds are low in net carbohydrates, as a large amount of their carbohydrate content is dietary fiber, which is not absorbed by the body. This makes them an intriguing alternative for people seeking to maintain ketosis while still benefiting from key nutrients.

In addition to being low in net carbohydrates, chia seeds are a great source of healthful lipids, including omega-3 fatty acids. These fats can add to the fat intake necessary for a ketogenic diet.

 Chia seeds also include a tiny quantity of protein, aiding in muscle upkeep and overall nourishment. Moreover, the high fiber content in chia seeds might induce a feeling of fullness, which may assist those on a ketogenic diet in controlling their appetite and preventing snacking between meals.

Chia seeds can be included in keto-friendly recipes, such as chia pudding, and low-carb smoothies, and as a thickening agent in sauces and soups. chia seeds offer a unique and varied choice for persons following a ketogenic diet, allowing them to retain their nutritional objectives while enjoying the myriad health benefits these seeds have to offer.

Chia Seeds In Special Diets

Chia seeds have gained substantial appeal in recent years, particularly for their versatility in addressing various dietary requirements. They are a great source of important nutrients, making them a perfect addition to special diets.

Whether you're following a gluten-free diet, a vegan or vegetarian lifestyle, focusing on athletic performance, or adhering to a ketogenic diet, chia seeds can play a crucial role in optimizing your nutrition.

Chia Seeds In Gluten-Free Diets

Chia seeds are innately gluten-free, making them a safe and healthful solution for anyone with celiac disease or gluten intolerance.

These tiny seeds can be used as a thickening ingredient in gluten-free baking, giving an ideal alternative to standard gluten-containing thickeners like flour or cornstarch. Chia seeds' propensity to absorb liquid and produce a gel-like consistency might assist in retaining the appropriate texture in gluten-free dishes while giving a boost of fiber, omega-3 fatty acids, and protein.

Chia Seeds In Vegan And Vegetarian Diets

Chia seeds are a plant-based powerhouse of nutrients, making them a great supplement to vegan and vegetarian diets.

These seeds are a fantastic source of protein, supplying all essential amino acids, which can be particularly advantageous for people seeking alternate protein sources.

Moreover, chia seeds are rich in omega-3 fatty acids, vital for heart and brain health, and they can be used as an egg alternative in vegan baking due to their propensity to bind components together. Chia seeds also give vital minerals, such as calcium and iron, which might be especially useful for persons not ingesting dairy or animal products.

CHAPTER SIX

Safety And Potential Side Effects Of Chia Seeds Supplement

Chia seeds have gained popularity in recent years as a healthful and adaptable nutritional supplement. These small seeds, originating from the Salvia hispanica plant, are rich in critical nutrients, such as omega-3 fatty acids, fiber, and protein. While they offer several health benefits, it is necessary to be aware of potential safety considerations and side effects related to their usage.

Allergies And Chia Seeds

One of the biggest safety concerns associated with chia seeds is the likelihood of allergies. While rare, some individuals may be allergic to chia seeds, resulting in severe effects. Allergic symptoms can vary from moderate to severe and may include itching, hives, swelling, or in more severe cases, anaphylaxis. It is crucial to be cautious if you have a known seed or nut allergy and to check with a healthcare expert before integrating chia seeds into your diet. Always start with a tiny dosage to monitor any potential allergic responses.

Choking Hazards And Chia Seeds

Chia seeds have a particular feature that might cause a choking threat when not swallowed properly. When exposed to liquid, they can absorb it and produce a gel-like substance.

This feature can be useful in some culinary applications, such as making chia pudding, but it can be harmful if not managed carefully.

In their dry state, chia seeds are small and firm, making them simple to inhale or swallow without chewing.

To prevent choking, it is recommended to soak chia seeds before swallowing them or mix them well with a sufficient amount of liquid. Children and others with swallowing issues should be extremely cautious when using chia seeds.

Chia Seeds And Medication Interactions

Chia seeds may interact with some drugs due to their unique composition. Notably, chia seeds are abundant in dietary fiber, which can slow down the absorption of several medications in the digestive tract.

This can be useful for regulating blood sugar levels and minimizing the risk of digestive difficulties, but it may also impair the absorption of drugs. If you are taking prescription medications, particularly ones with specific scheduling requirements, it is advised to visit your healthcare professional to discuss potential interactions and the optimum time of chia seed use. Adjustments to medication schedules may be necessary to ensure the drugs' effectiveness.

while chia seeds are regarded as a nutritional and health-promoting supplement, it is vital to be aware of potential safety concerns and side effects related to their usage.

 Allergies to chia seeds can develop, and persons with documented seed or nut allergies should exercise caution. Choking concerns are prevalent when chia seeds are not sufficiently soaked in liquid, making correct preparation crucial. Moreover, persons taking prescription medications should consult their healthcare professionals to identify potential interactions and guarantee their medication's effectiveness. By being aware and cautious, consumers can enjoy the many benefits of chia seeds while limiting any hazards.

Buying And Storing Chia Seeds

Chia seeds have gained enormous popularity in recent years due to their nutritional benefits and adaptability in numerous recipes. When it comes to introducing chia seeds into your diet, it's necessary to consider both the buying procedure and correct storage to ensure their quality and freshness.

Choosing The Best Quality Chia Seeds

Selecting high-quality chia seeds is vital to maximize the nutritional benefits they give. Here are some aspects to consider while buying chia seeds:

hue and Appearance: High-quality chia seeds should have a uniform, dark hue, usually ranging from black to brown. Avoid seeds with a mottled or discolored look, as this may suggest rotting or inferior quality.

Smell: Chia seeds should have a pleasant, nutty fragrance. If they have a sour or off-putting scent, it's better to avoid them, as this can be an indication of oxidation.

packing: Check the packing for any evidence of damage or manipulation. Chia seeds are often sold in sealed, resealable bags or containers to retain freshness. Ensure that the packing is intact to prevent exposure to air and moisture.

Certifications: Look for chia seeds that have been certified as organic, non-GMO, or by a trustworthy quality control agency. These certifications can imply a better level of quality and purity.

Reputation of the Brand: Opt for chia seeds from renowned brands or sources with positive customer evaluations. This can provide some assurance of quality.

Origin: Chia seeds are native to South America, therefore seeds purchased from regions like Mexico, Argentina, or Bolivia are frequently of good quality. Be cautious of the source and provenance of the chia seeds you purchase.

Proper Storage To Maintain Freshness

To retain the freshness and shelf life of chia seeds, careful storage is vital. Chia seeds have natural oils that can grow rancid when exposed to heat, light, and moisture. Here are some rules for keeping chia seeds:

Airtight Container: Once you've opened the original packing, move the chia seeds to an airtight container. This helps prevent air and moisture from damaging the seeds.

Cool and Dark Place: Store the container in a cool, dark place, such as a pantry or cupboard. Avoid exposing the seeds to direct sunlight or heat sources, as this might expedite the deterioration of their natural oils.

chilling: While not necessary, chilling can extend the shelf life of chia seeds, especially in warmer and more humid locations. If you wish to refrigerate them, ensure they are in an airtight container to prevent moisture absorption.

Freezing: Chia seeds can also be frozen, which considerably prolongs their shelf life.

Divide them into smaller parts and store them in airtight bags or containers in the freezer. Freezing is a fantastic choice for long-term storage.

Regular Checks: Periodically examine the chia seeds for any signs of deterioration, such as an off scent or peculiar color. If you find any difficulties, it's better to toss them and replace them with fresh seeds.

purchasing high-quality chia seeds and keeping them properly are crucial steps to ensure you get the most out of this healthy supplement. By considering elements like look, scent, packaging, and origin when purchasing chia seeds, and following the prescribed storage instructions, you may enjoy their health benefits and culinary diversity for an extended period.

CHAPTER SEVEN

Chia Seeds In Traditional And Indigenous Medicine

Chia seeds have a deep history in traditional and indigenous medicine, with their use extending back thousands of years. Indigenous people across the Americas, particularly in places like Mexico, Central America, and South America, have recognized the nutritional and therapeutic potential of chia seeds. These tiny seeds were treasured for their capacity to give food and offer different health advantages.

Chia Seeds In Indigenous Healing Practices

Chia seeds are a valuable medicinal resource that has been used extensively in indigenous healing techniques.

Several health issues were addressed by consuming the seeds.

For example, indigenous people employed chia seeds, which were well-known for their hydrating qualities, as a source of water during lengthy walks or physically demanding tasks. Chia seeds combine to create a gel-like substance that can aid in retaining moisture and warding off dehydration.

Additionally, chia seeds were utilized to reduce gastrointestinal pain. Their high fiber content functioned as a natural constipation treatment and improved digestion. Furthermore, it was believed that chia seeds had anti-inflammatory qualities, which made them useful for treating inflammatory diseases like arthritis.

Chia seeds were used as a traditional energy source in some indigenous civilizations. To increase their energy and endurance before battle, Aztec warriors, for instance, would eat chia seeds. These age-old customs emphasize the rich nutritional content of the seeds and their significance for maintaining both physical and mental health.

Chia Seeds' Folklore And Cultural Significance

Indigenous tribes place a great deal of cultural and folkloric significance on chia seeds. Chia seeds were employed in religious ceremonies and rituals and were regarded as a sacred meal in many indigenous societies. It was thought that the seeds had a mystical significance and represented fertility, life, and rebirth.

Because chia seeds are abundant in oil and contain important fatty acids like omega-3, the word "chia" itself comes from the Nahuatl word "chian," which means "oily." The ability of the seeds to support and nurture life was acknowledged by indigenous populations, who also gave them legendary characteristics.

Chia seeds are associated with creation myths and the universe's beginnings in some native cultures. They were regarded as a gift from the gods, and eating them was thought to facilitate communication with the divine. Chia seeds, which stand for prosperity and abundance, were also offered in a variety of ceremonies.

Chia seeds are still cherished today due to their cultural importance and health advantages. Because of their exceptional dietary profile—which includes fiber, protein, omega-3 fatty acids, and antioxidants—they have gained popularity as a superfood on a global scale. People are honoring the indigenous cultures that have shared and conserved their knowledge of this remarkable seed for decades, as more and more people become aware of the nutritional benefits of chia seeds.

CHAPTER EIGHT

Chia Seeds And Upcoming Studies

Chia seeds' abundance of omega-3 fatty acids, dietary fiber, and other important elements has made them a highly sought-after nutritional supplement.

Still, there are a ton of directions that might be explored in the future for chia seed research because the area is far from full. Our knowledge of chia seeds and their possible health advantages is expected to grow as a result of these ongoing research projects and future discoveries.

The effect of chia seeds on cardiovascular health is one topic of interest for further study. Chia seeds are recognized for their high content of alpha-linolenic acid (ALA), an omega-3 fatty acid derived from plants.

Lower blood pressure and improved cholesterol are two heart disease risk factors that have been linked to ALA. Further research on these pathways and the long-term impacts of chia seed consumption on heart health may be conducted in the future.

Moreover, antioxidants, which are essential for shielding cells from oxidative damage, are abundant in chia seeds.

Subsequent investigations may examine the possible role of chia seeds in mitigating oxidative stress inside the human body, hence reducing the likelihood of chronic ailments like diabetes and cancer.

Examining the precise kinds and concentrations of antioxidants in chia seeds as well as how bioavailable they are to the human body may yield important information.

The high fiber content of chia seeds is another well-known benefit that helps facilitate digestion and increase feelings of fullness. The impact of chia seeds on gut health and gut flora could be the subject of this research. Comprehensive knowledge of the effects of chia seeds on the diversity and makeup of the gut microbiota may have profound effects on general health and well-being.

Furthermore, the possible benefit of chia seeds for controlling weight is gaining attention. According to certain research, chia seeds may aid in hunger regulation and weight loss. Subsequent studies could examine the fundamental processes underlying these outcomes and evaluate the long-term viability of utilizing chia seeds as a dietary supplement for weight control.

Current Research And Possible Findings
Research is still being done to better understand the many health advantages and possible uses of chia seeds.

Scholars are now investigating several facets of chia seeds, such as their physiological impacts, nutritional makeup, and bioavailability.

To acquire a thorough grasp of the topic, these investigations frequently incorporate controlled experiments, clinical trials, and epidemiological research.

The bioavailability of the nutrients in chia seeds is one topic of continuing study. Calcium, magnesium, and phosphorus are among the vital elements found in chia seeds; however, some of these minerals are confined within the seed's structure. Research is looking into ways to increase these nutrients' bioavailability so that the body can absorb them more easily. The findings of this study may have consequences for treating mineral deficiencies in people whose access to a variety of food sources is restricted.

Research on how chia seeds affect blood sugar management is another facet of ongoing investigations. Chia seeds may help regulate blood sugar levels, which can be especially helpful for people who already have diabetes or are at risk of getting the disease, according to some preliminary research. The goal of ongoing research is to identify the ideal dosage for glycemic management as well as to clarify the processes underlying these benefits.

Research is also being done on chia seeds' ability to reduce inflammation. Numerous medical disorders, such as arthritis, cancer, and cardiovascular disease, are associated with chronic inflammation.

Because chia seeds are a rich source of antioxidants and omega-3 fatty acids, researchers are investigating whether consuming them can help lower inflammation markers in the body. If verified, this may create new avenues for the treatment and prevention of inflammatory illnesses.

Conclusion

Because of its exceptional nutritional profile and possible health benefits, chia seeds have drawn the interest of both researchers and health enthusiasts. There is still a lot to learn about the benefits of chia seeds for digestive health, weight loss, and cardiovascular health, even though much has already been learned.

Subsequent investigations may reveal the complex processes via which chia seeds influence different facets of human health. Chia seeds offer a plethora of prospects for additional research, ranging from gut microbiota and anti-inflammatory effects to cardiovascular health and antioxidant qualities.

In addition to advancing our understanding of chia seeds, these current research and prospective findings could result in the development of novel dietary plans and medical treatments that enhance human health and well-being.

It seems likely that chia seeds' status as a superfood will further increase as science works to solve its many riddles.